A SEASON OF MEMORIES

WINTER

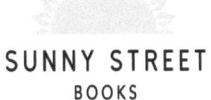

SUNNY STREET
BOOKS

Copyright © 2019 Sunny Street Books
All rights reserved.

"Once so much snow fell that my school was called off. I was so excited. A snow day! My brothers and I put on our warmest winter coats, along with our hats and mittens. Then we went outside and built the best snowman ever."

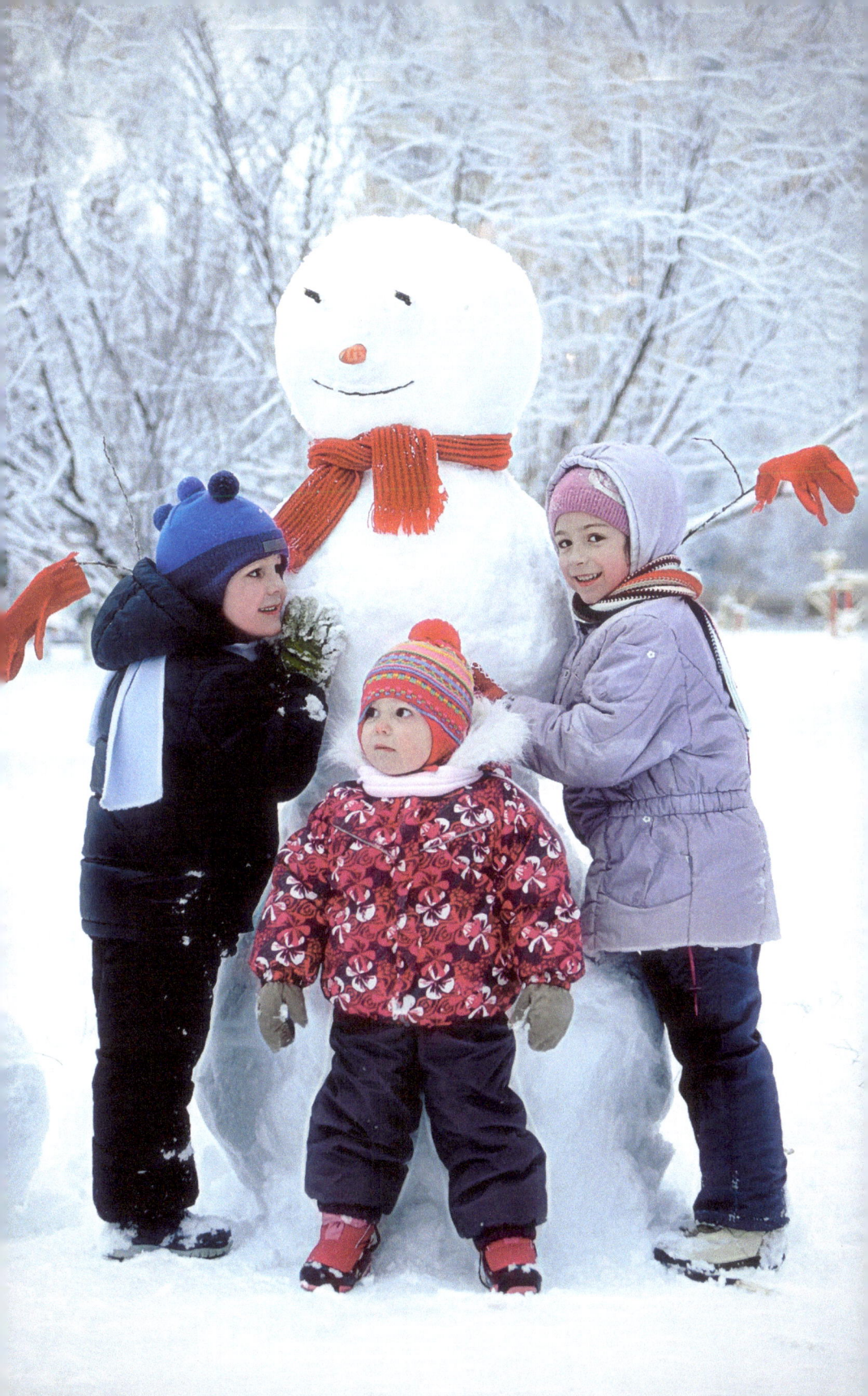

"When I was little, I wondered what snowflakes tasted like. So the next time it snowed, I stood outside with my mouth open. A few snowflakes landed on my tongue. But before I could figure out what they tasted like, they were gone!"

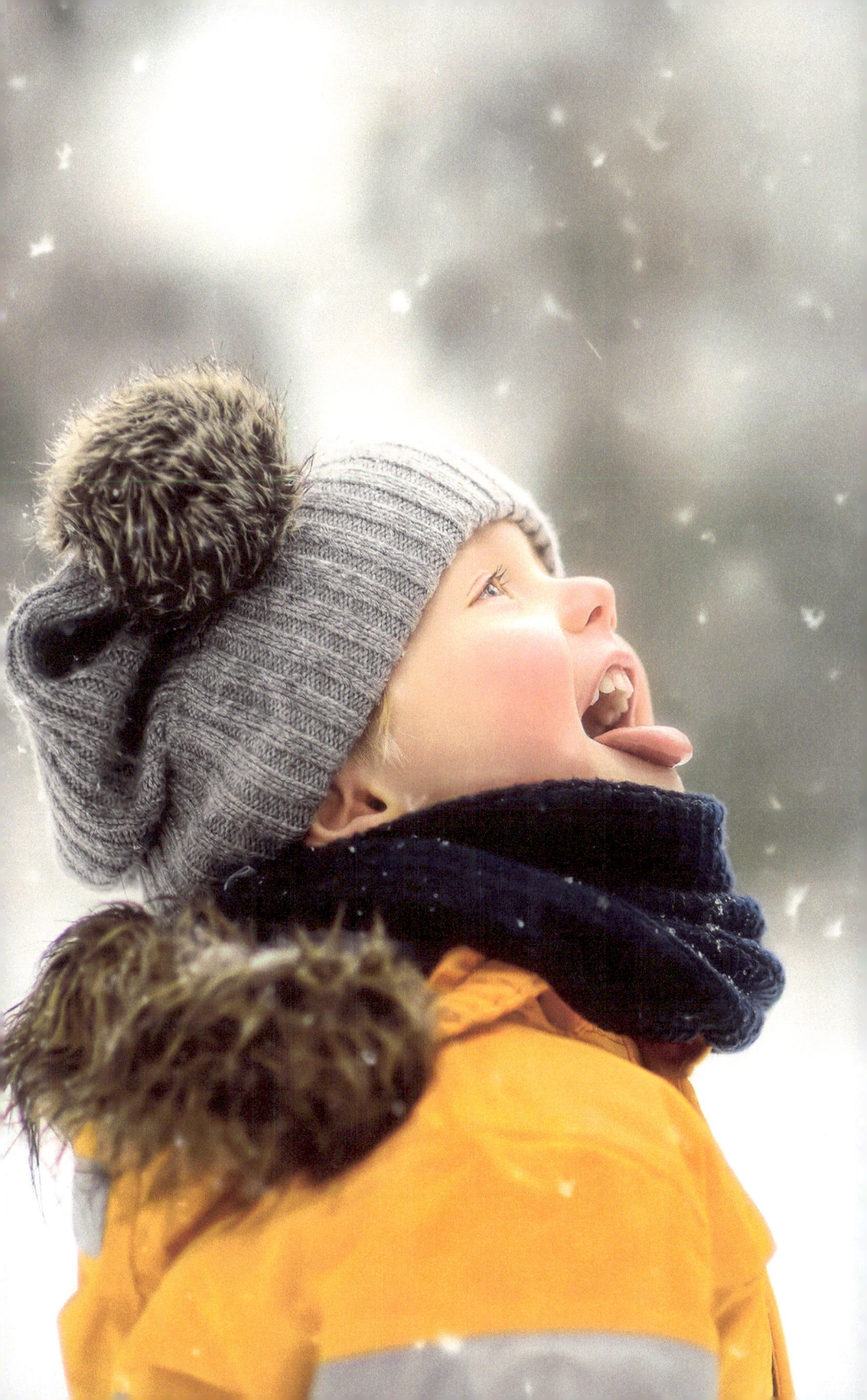

"There was a field behind our house that had a big hill. My brother and I couldn't wait for it to snow so we could go sledding. We didn't care how cold it was or how tired we got. We kept dragging our sled up that hill so we could slide down again."

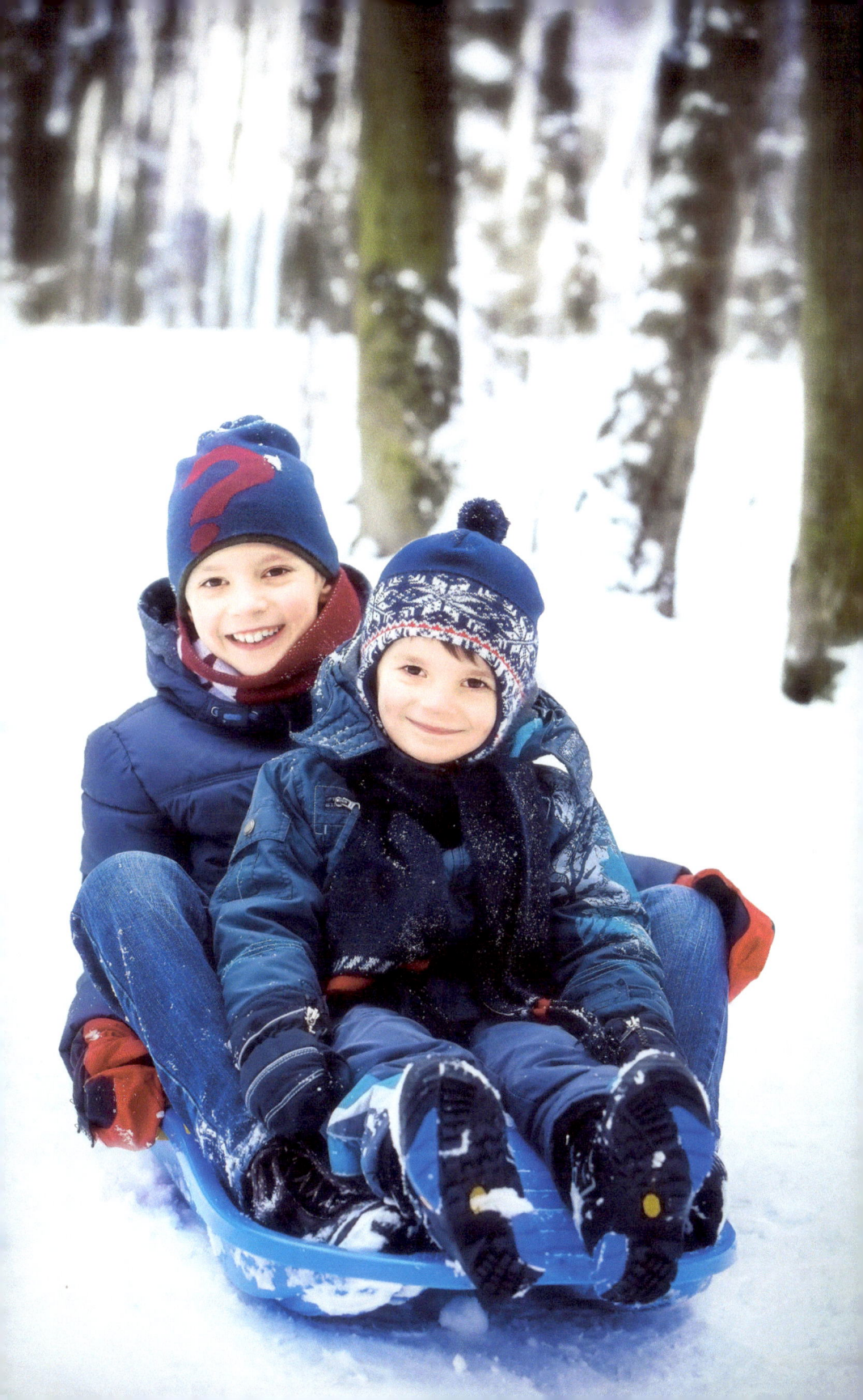

"I loved making paper snowflakes. I folded a piece of paper several times, cut it here and there, and when I opened it up, I had a snowflake. And just like real snowflakes, no two were ever alike."

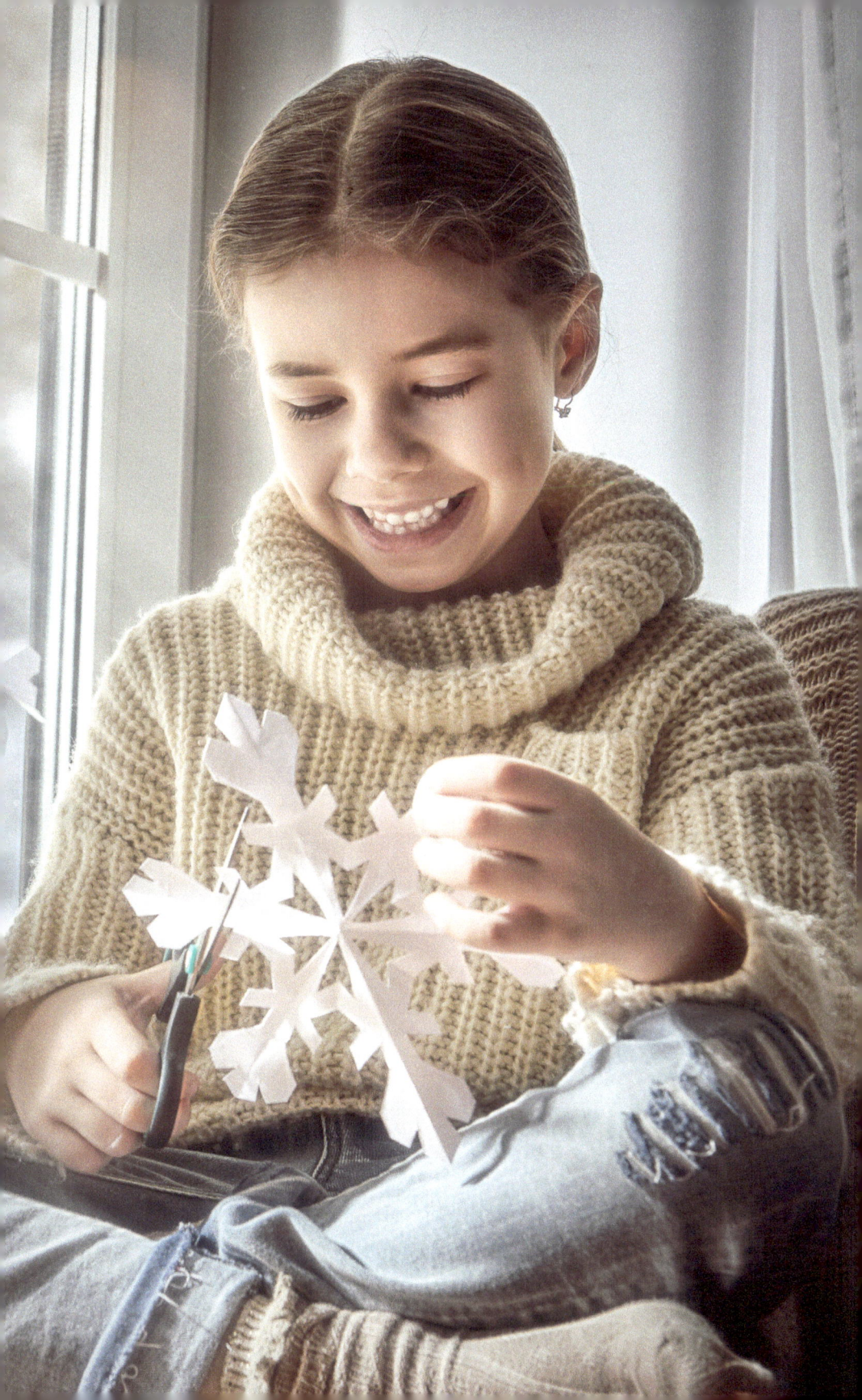

"One winter I worried that the birds in our backyard were cold and hungry. So my Mom helped me build a bird house, and we bought bird seed to go in it. The birds got so used to eating the seed that every time they saw me, they flew to the bird feeder."

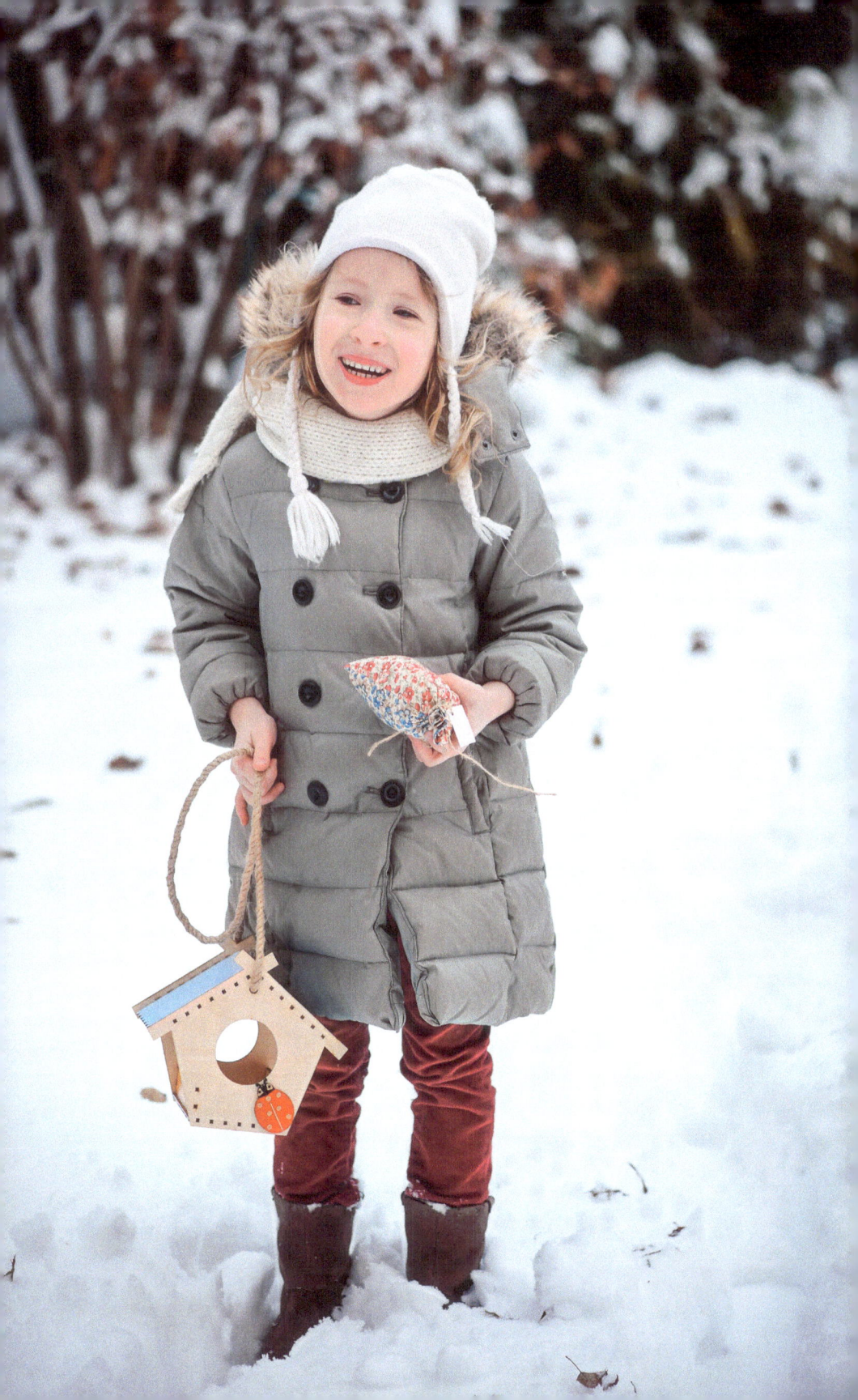

"My big sister told me that if I lay down in the snow and swished my arms and legs back and forth, I'd make a snow angel. I didn't believe her. But sure enough, when I stood up there was an angel in the snow."

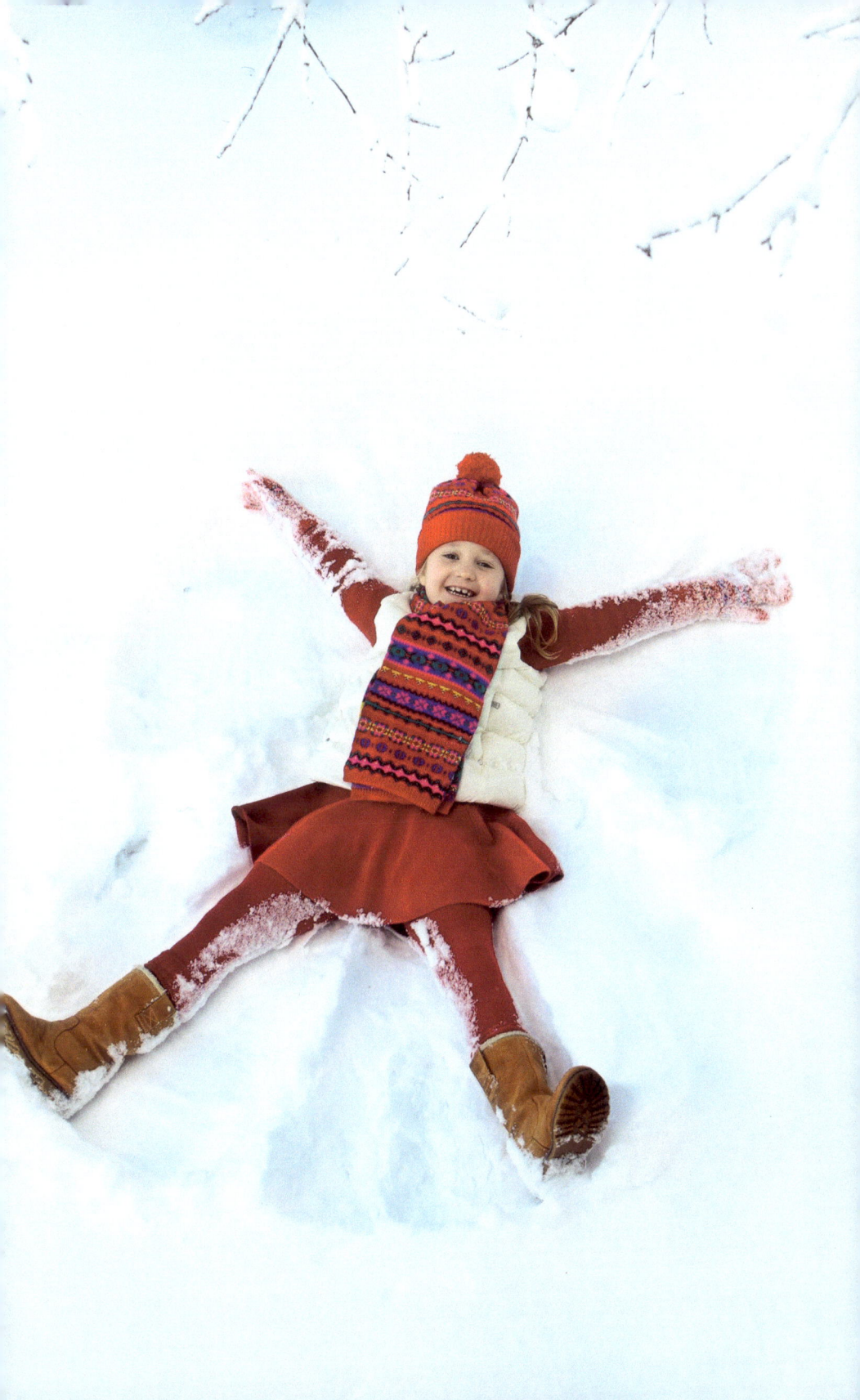

"When it was cold outside, I loved sitting on the window seat in my bedroom with my teddy bear and a cup of hot cocoa. Even though it was snowing outside, my room felt so warm and cozy."

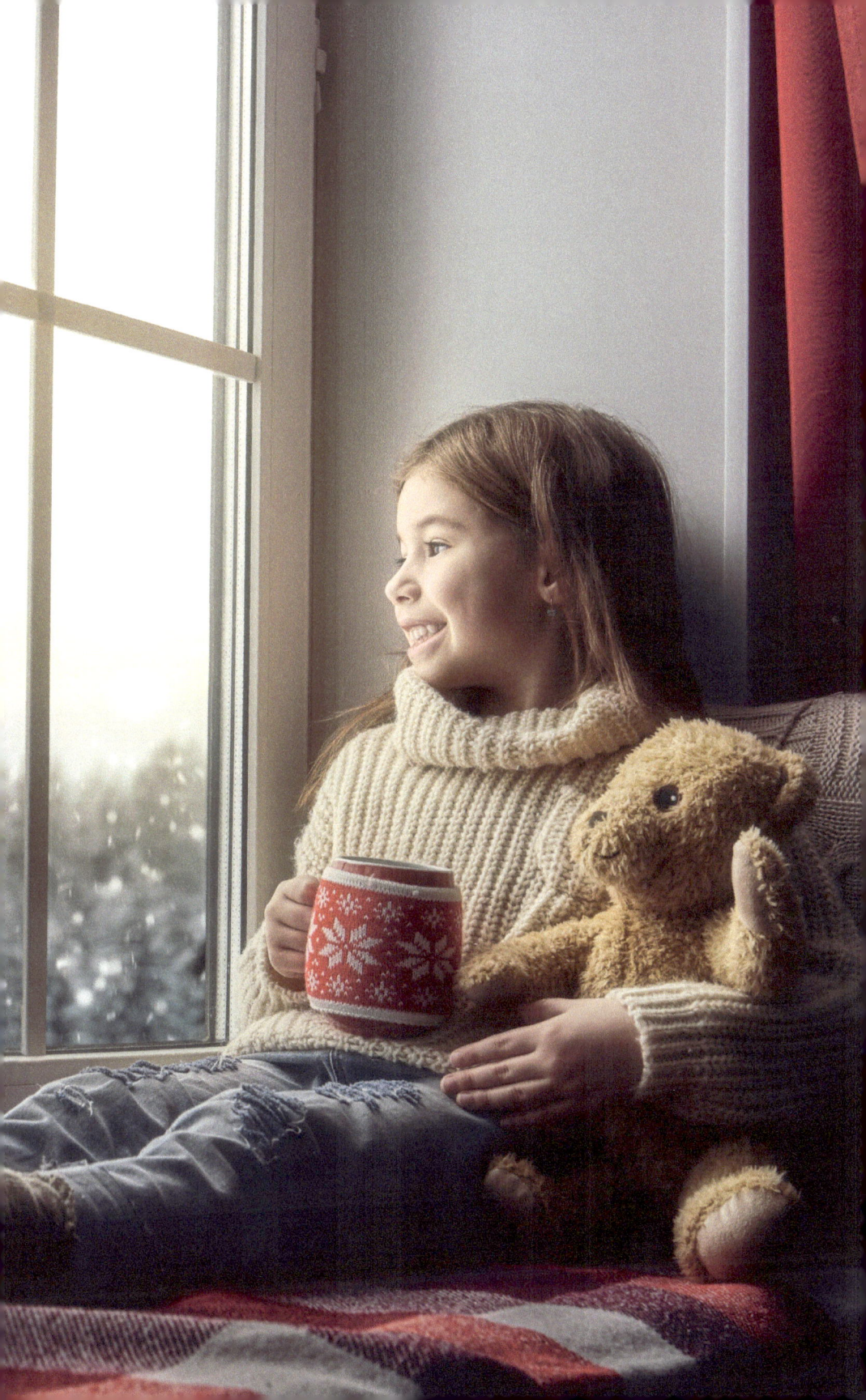

"There was an outdoor ice rink only a few blocks from our house. I loved ice skating more than anything, so I went there almost every day. As I twirled and glided, I pretended I was an Olympic ice skater going for a gold medal."

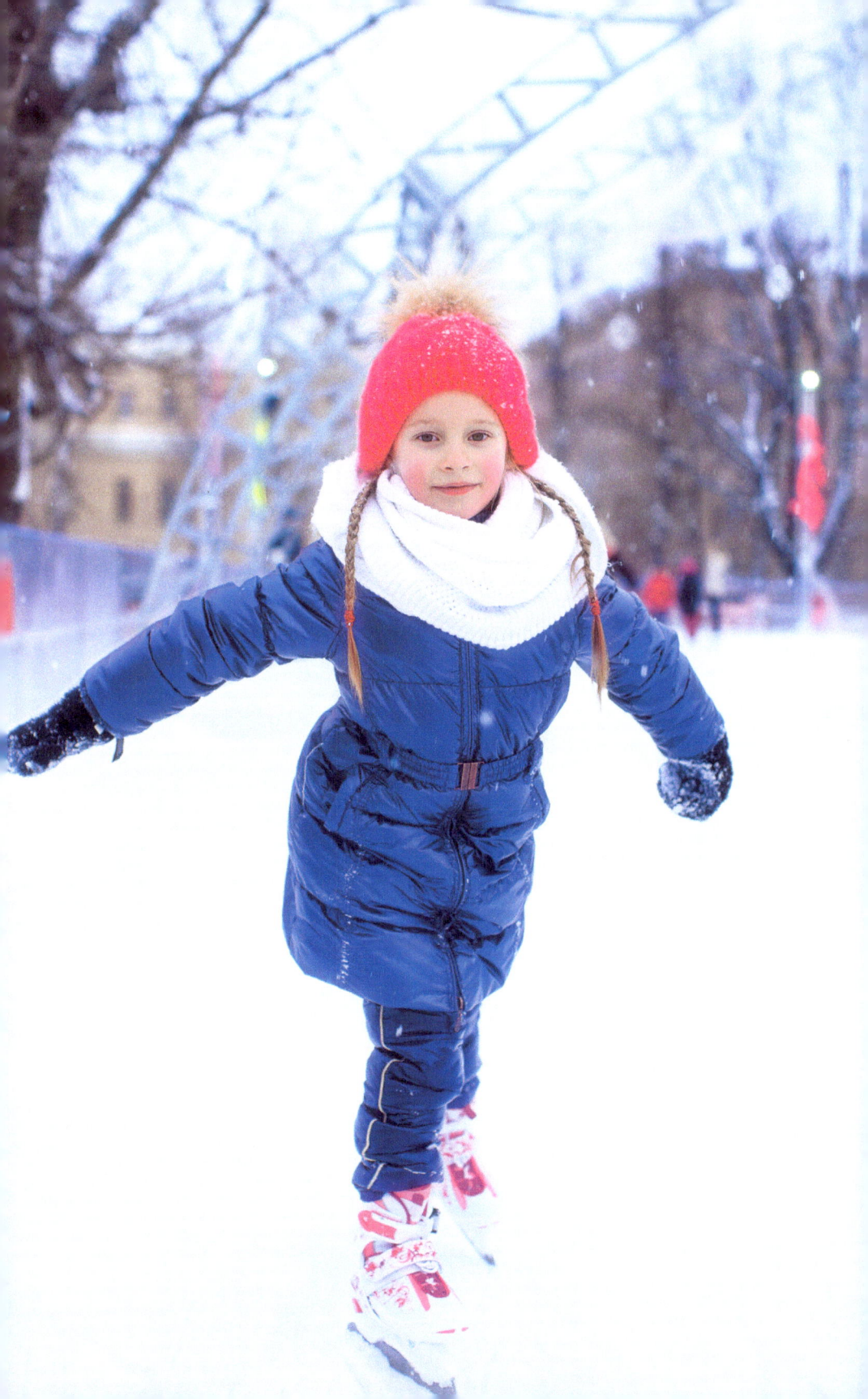

"Whenever it snowed, the first thing we did was go outside and have a snowball fight. We built snow forts to protect us and made snowballs for ammunition. We never really knew who won each battle. We just had fun doing it."

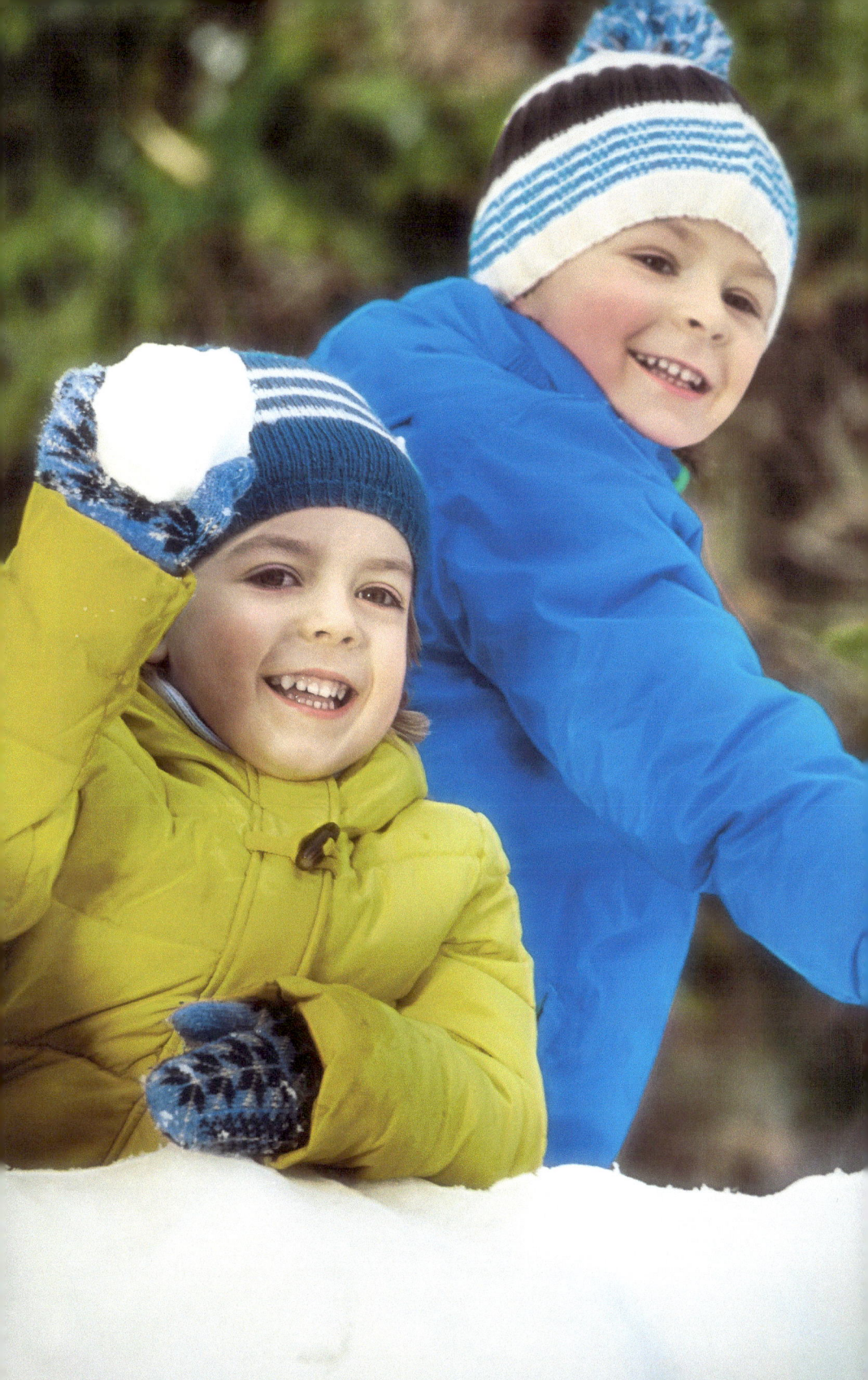

"Some mornings there was so much snow piled up on our car that it was hard to tell there was even a car under it! But I didn't mind. I loved holding the brush and *whooshing* the snow away."

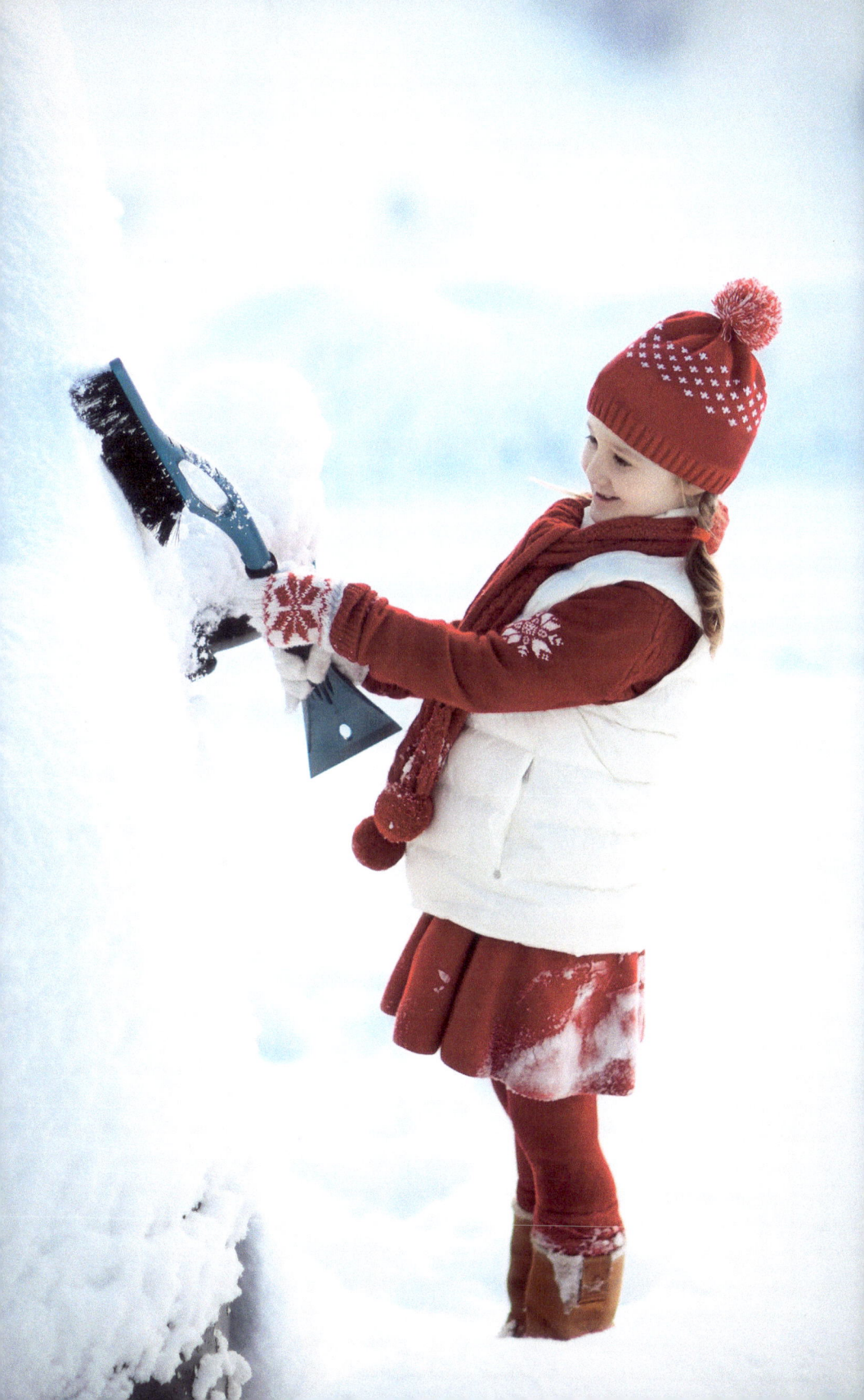

"One winter my family took a trip to the mountains, where I went skiing for the first time. At first I was scared, but I finally got the hang of it. By the end of our trip I was begging my parents to come back the next year."

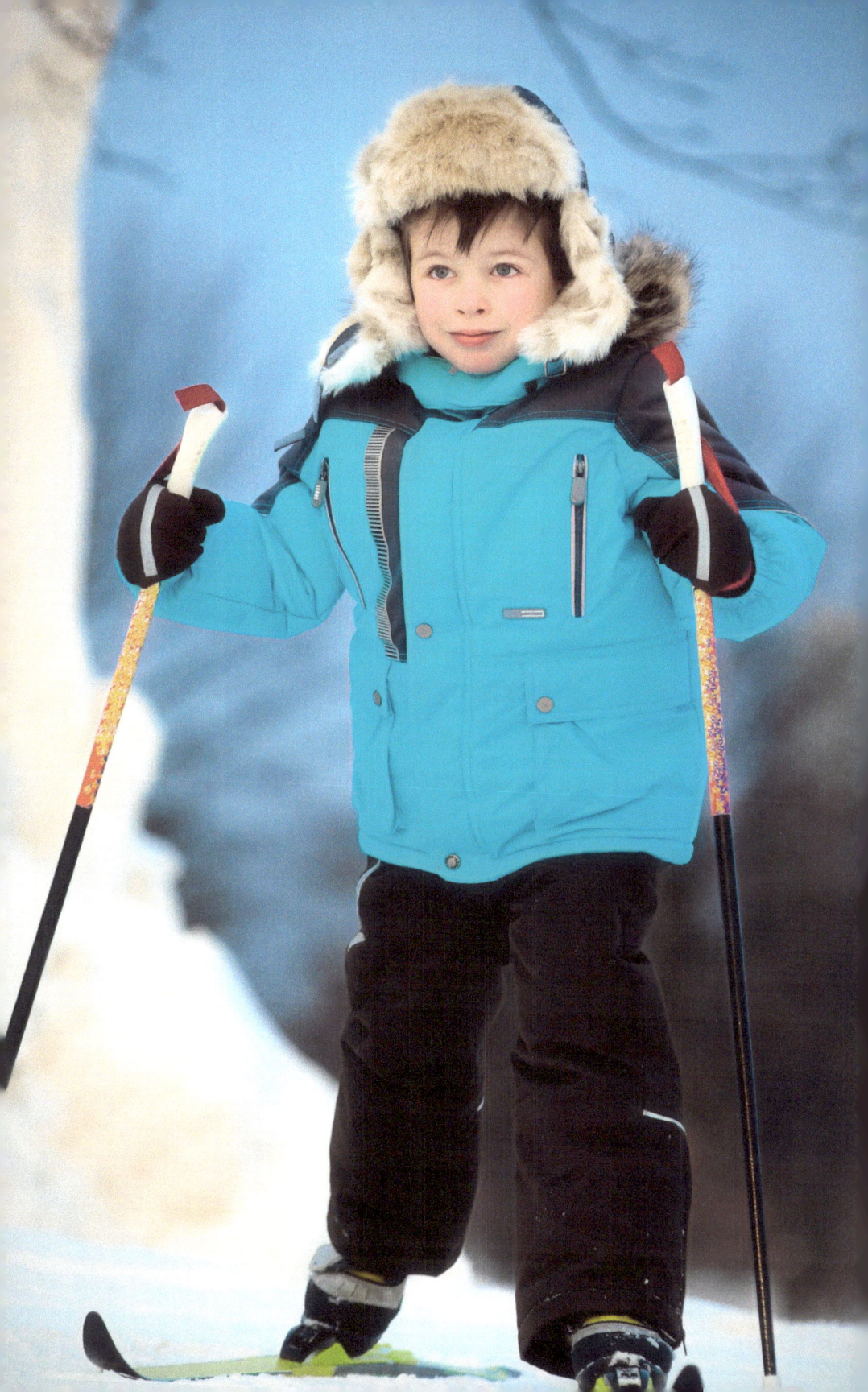

"In the winter, one of my jobs was shoveling snow off the sidewalk that led to our house. It was a lot of work, but it was worth it. Afterward my Mom always brought me inside and gave me cookies and hot cocoa."

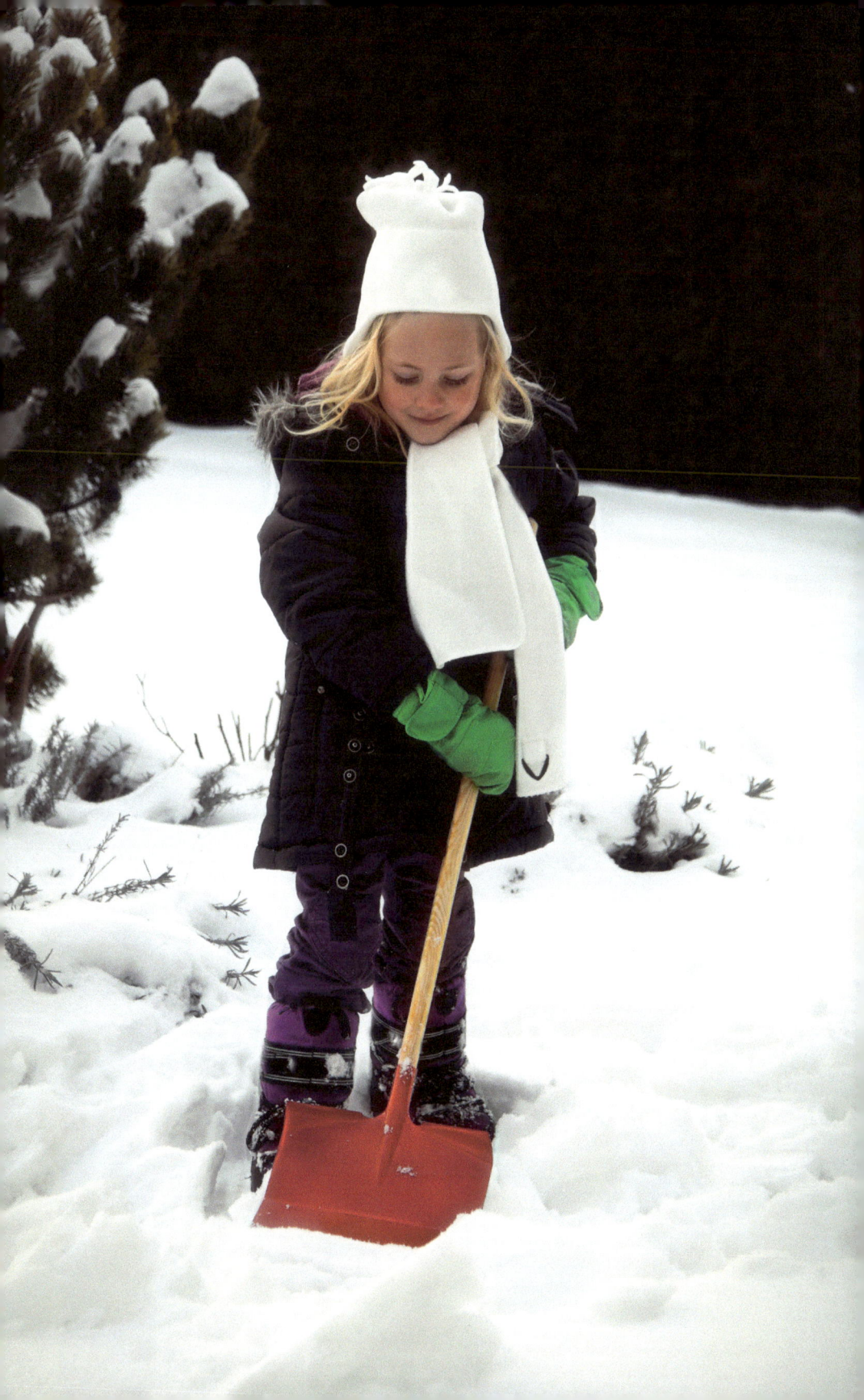

"I looked forward to winter weather every year just so I could put on my pink furry ear muffs. They were fun to wear at the same time they kept my ears toasty warm!"

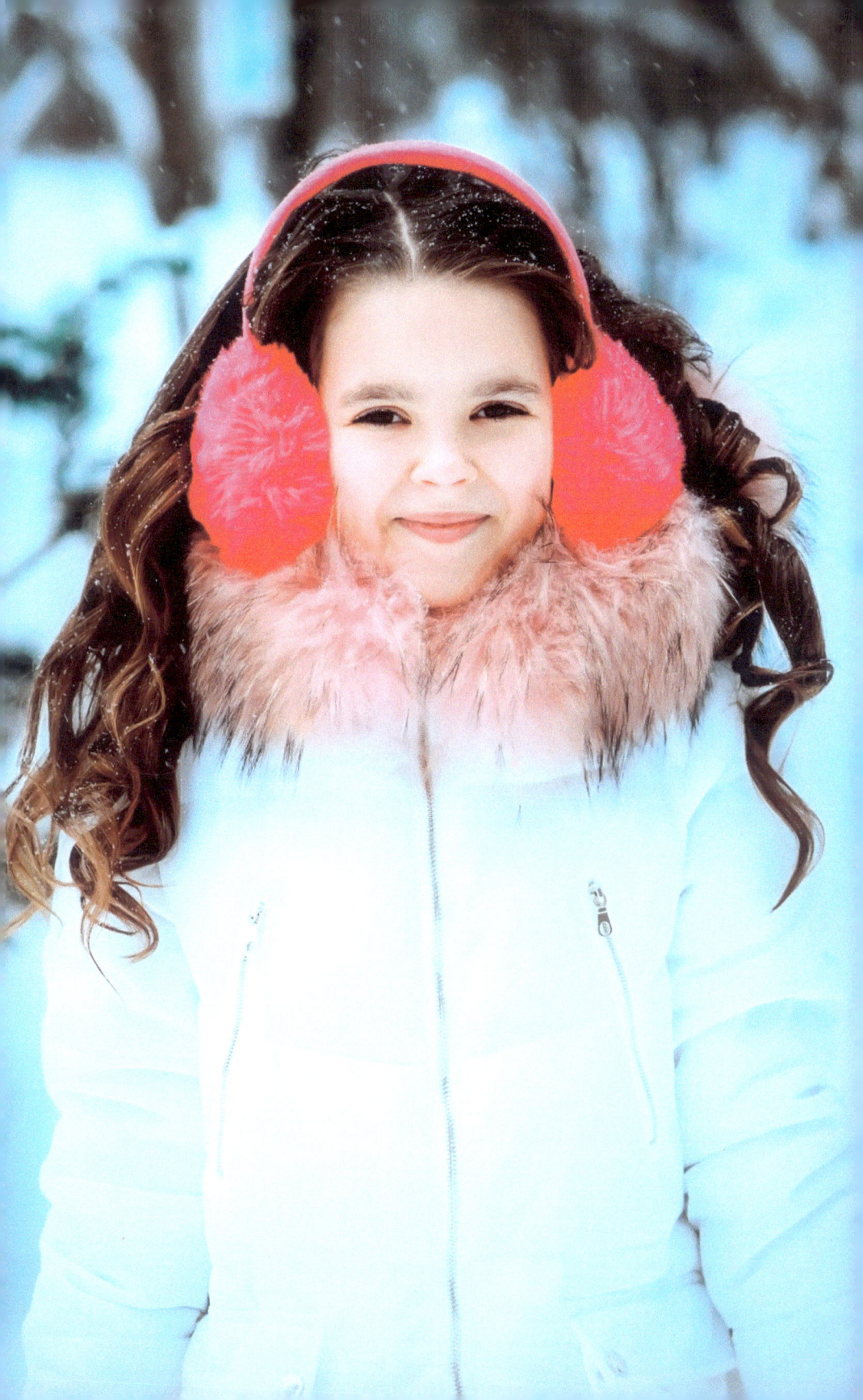

"One winter day I took a handful of nuts outside and waited near a tree. Pretty soon a squirrel scurried down the trunk. He came closer and closer. When he couldn't resist any longer, he finally took a nut right out of my hand."

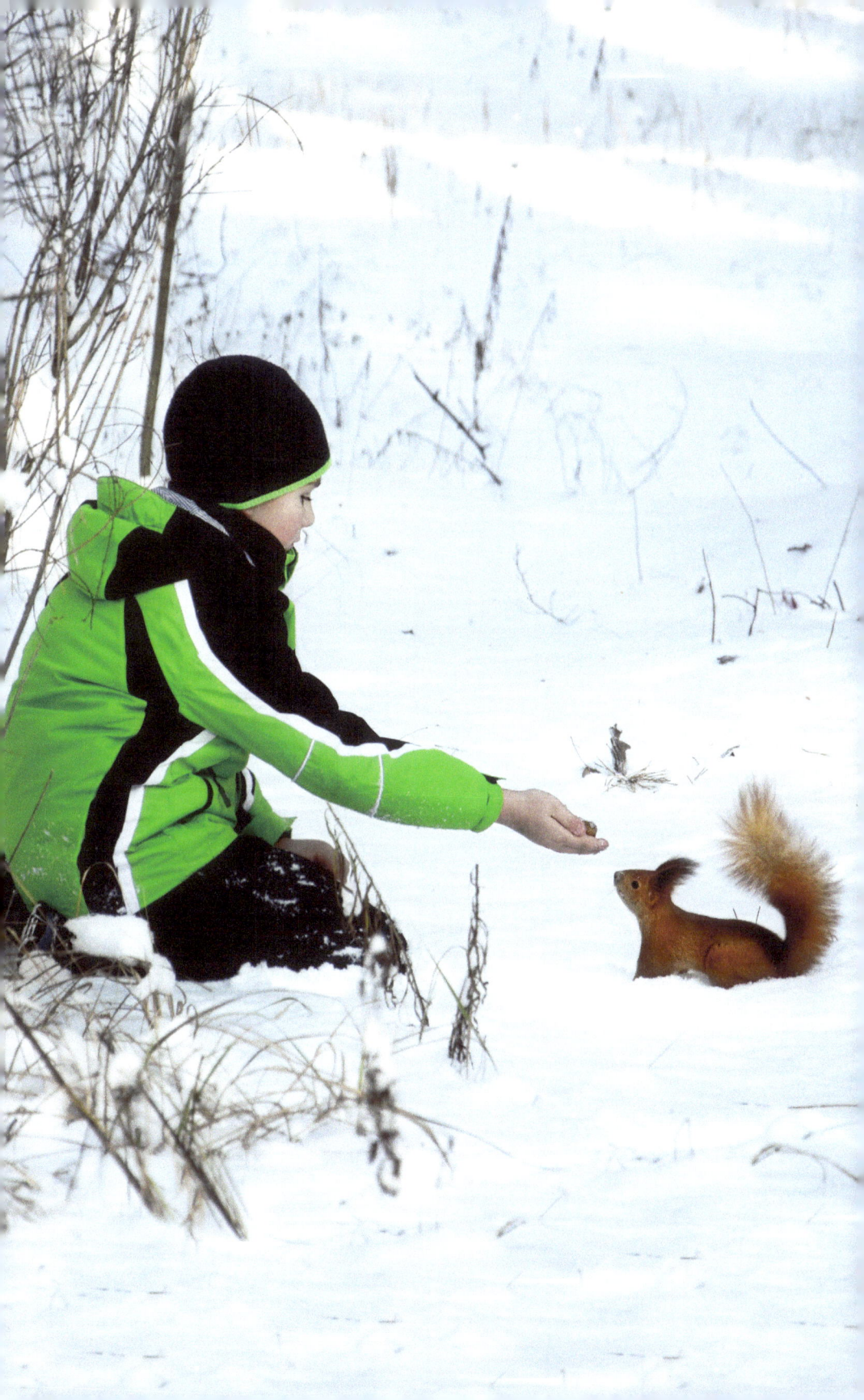

"Every year in the middle of December, we went to a Christmas tree lot to pick out our tree. Holiday music was always playing, and the wonderful scent of pine trees was everywhere. Just being there filled us with the spirit of Christmas."

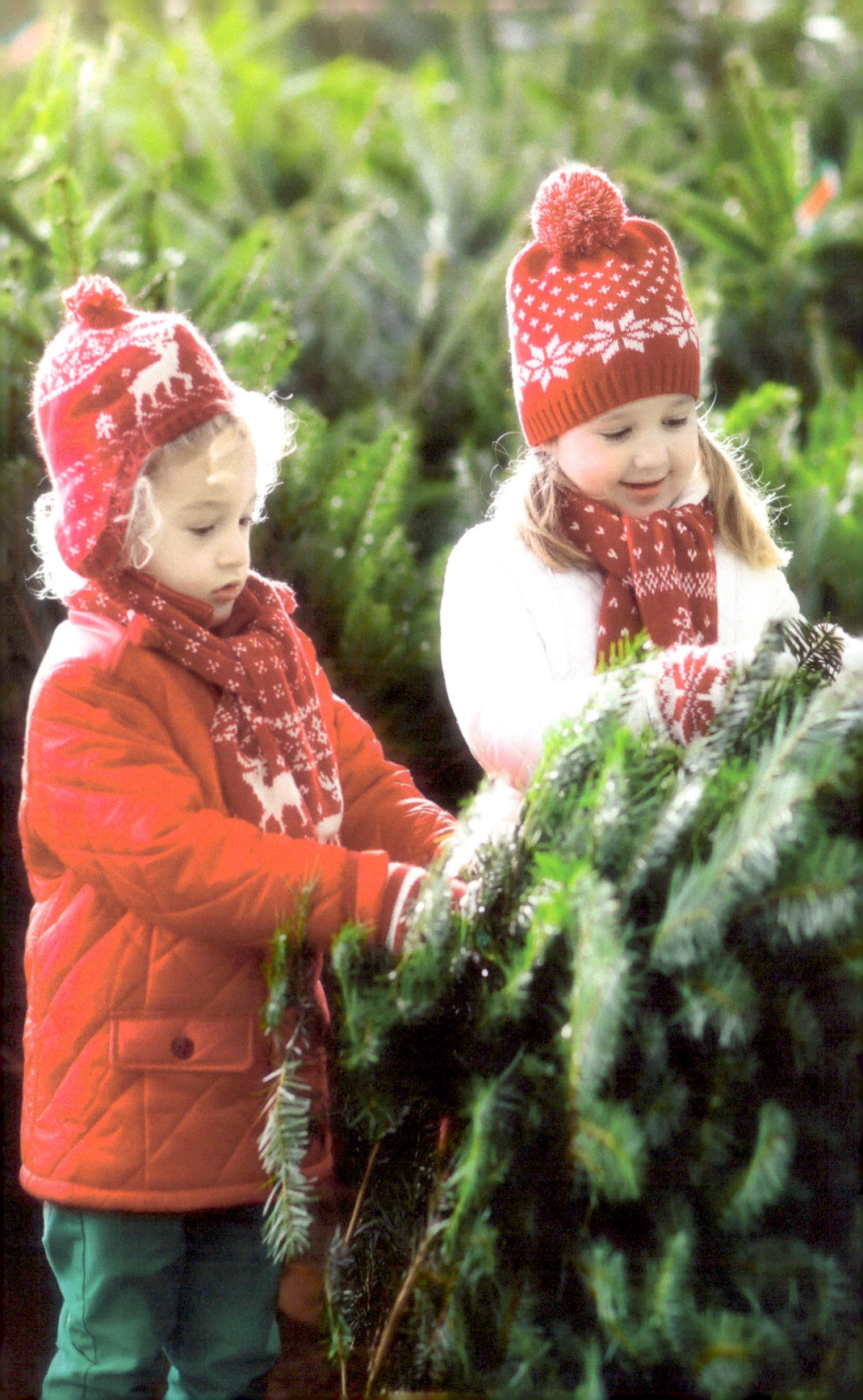

"Building a gingerbread house with my Mom was my favorite holiday activity. But even better than building it was eating it on Christmas day!"

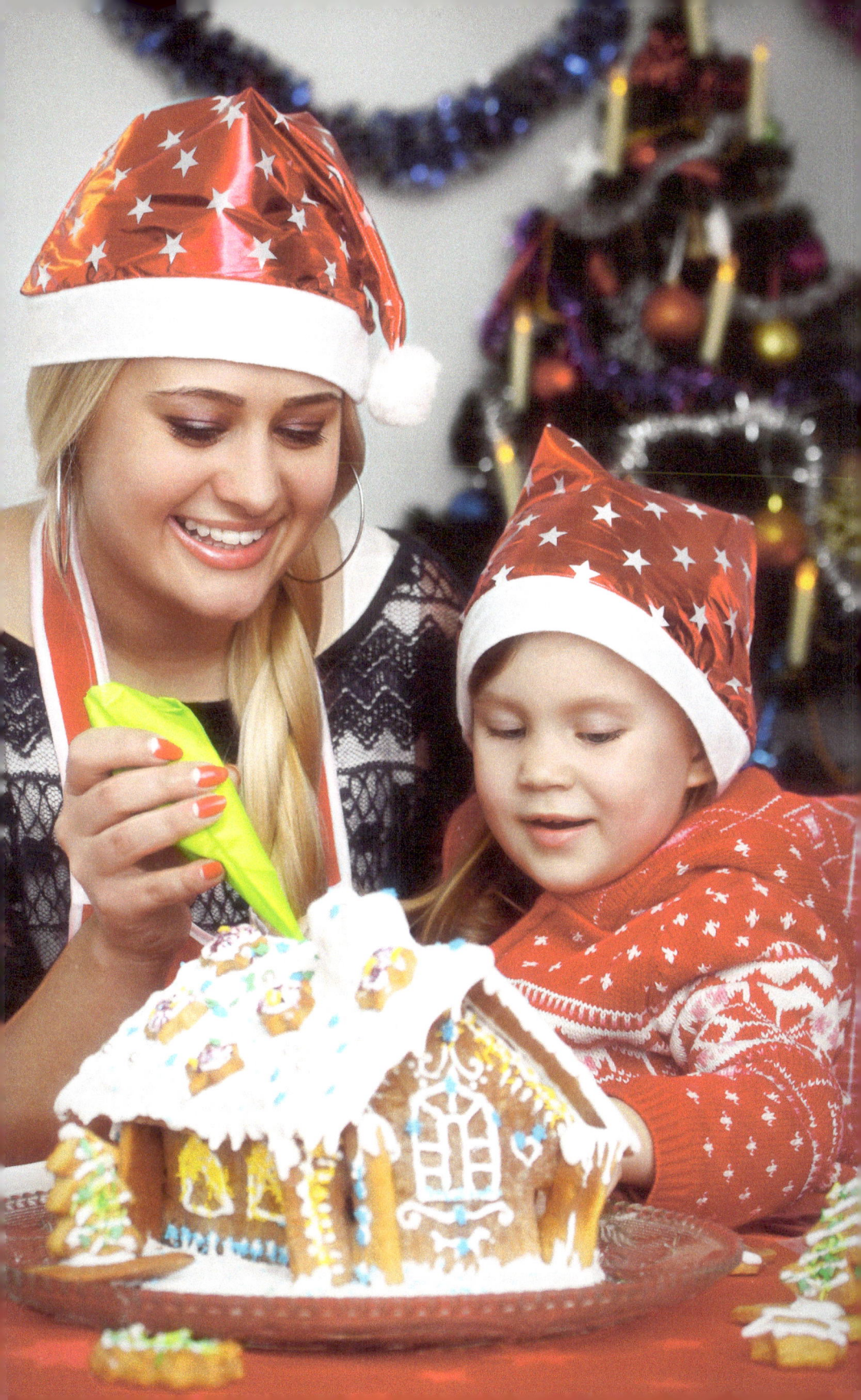

"My Mom once gave me a snow globe she had when she was a little girl. It was the first decoration I took out every holiday season. I couldn't wait to turn it upside down so I could watch the snow fall inside that tiny winter wonderland."

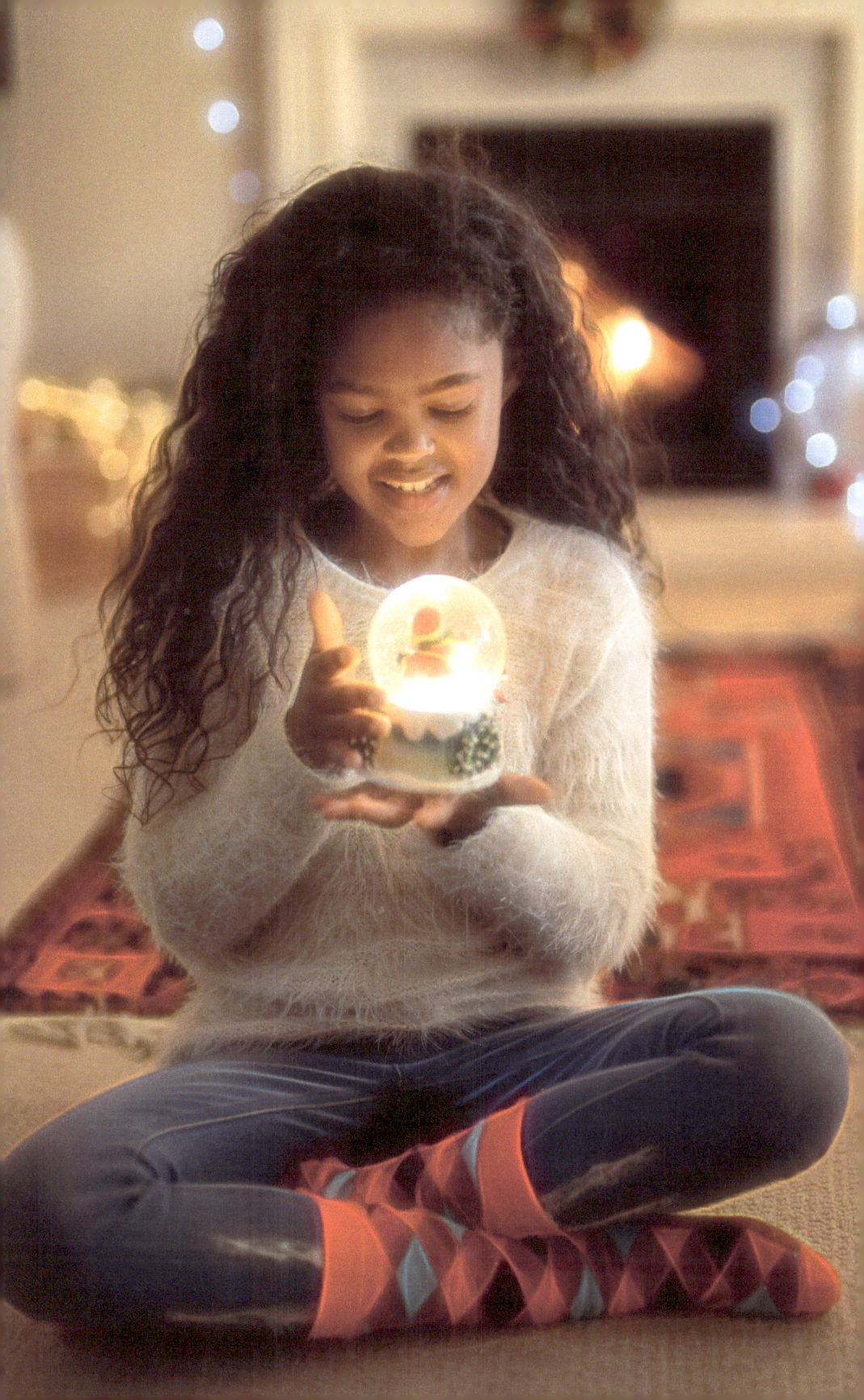

"I loved twinkling Christmas lights, the scent of pine and cinnamon, and the anticipation I felt that Santa would be coming soon. Every breath I took seemed to be filled with the wonder of Christmas."

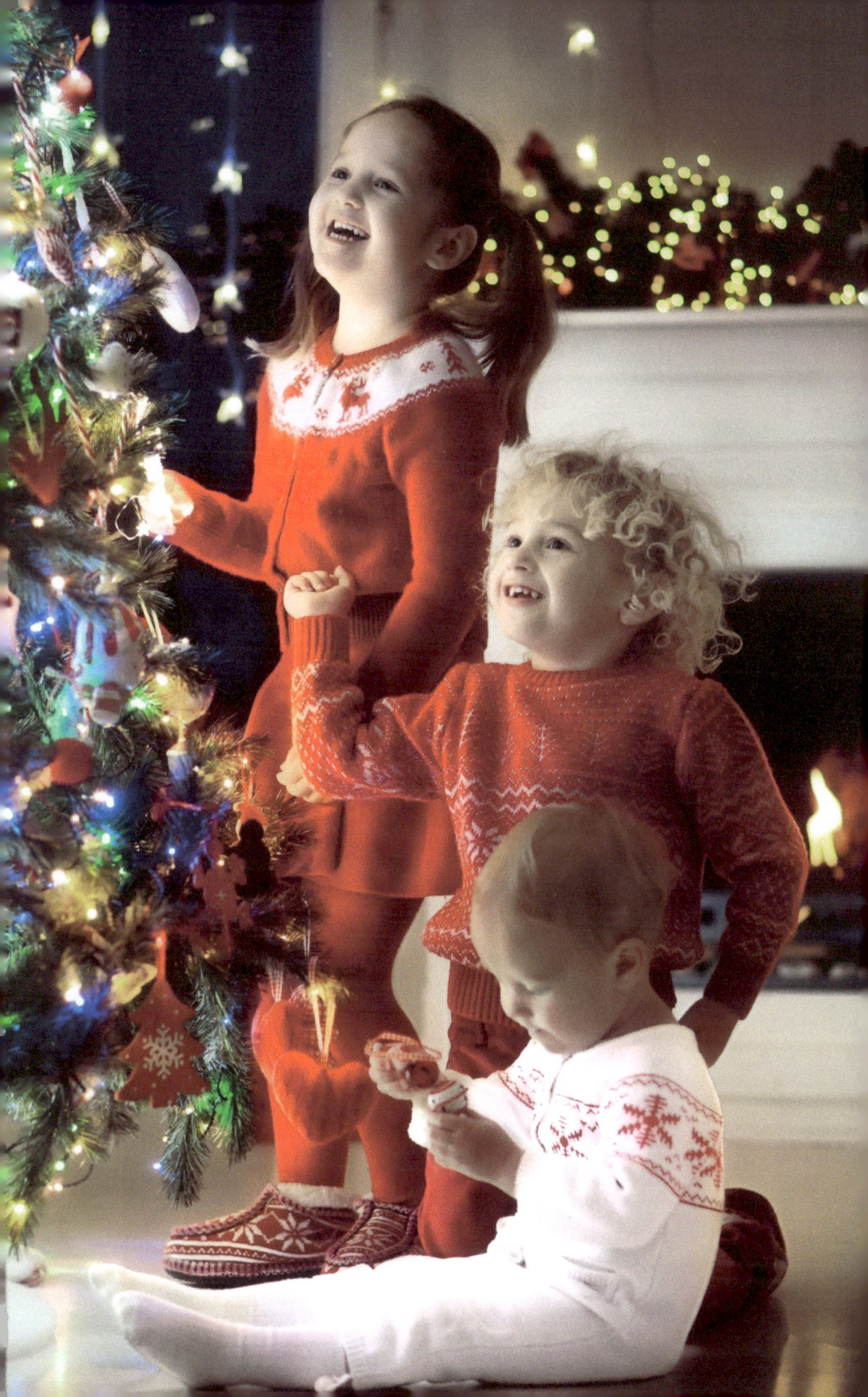

"One Christmas Eve, I decided to stay awake to meet Santa Claus. I lay on the floor and put his milk and cookies next to me so I wouldn't miss him. The next thing I knew, it was Christmas morning. The milk and cookies were gone, and Santa had left presents under the tree!"

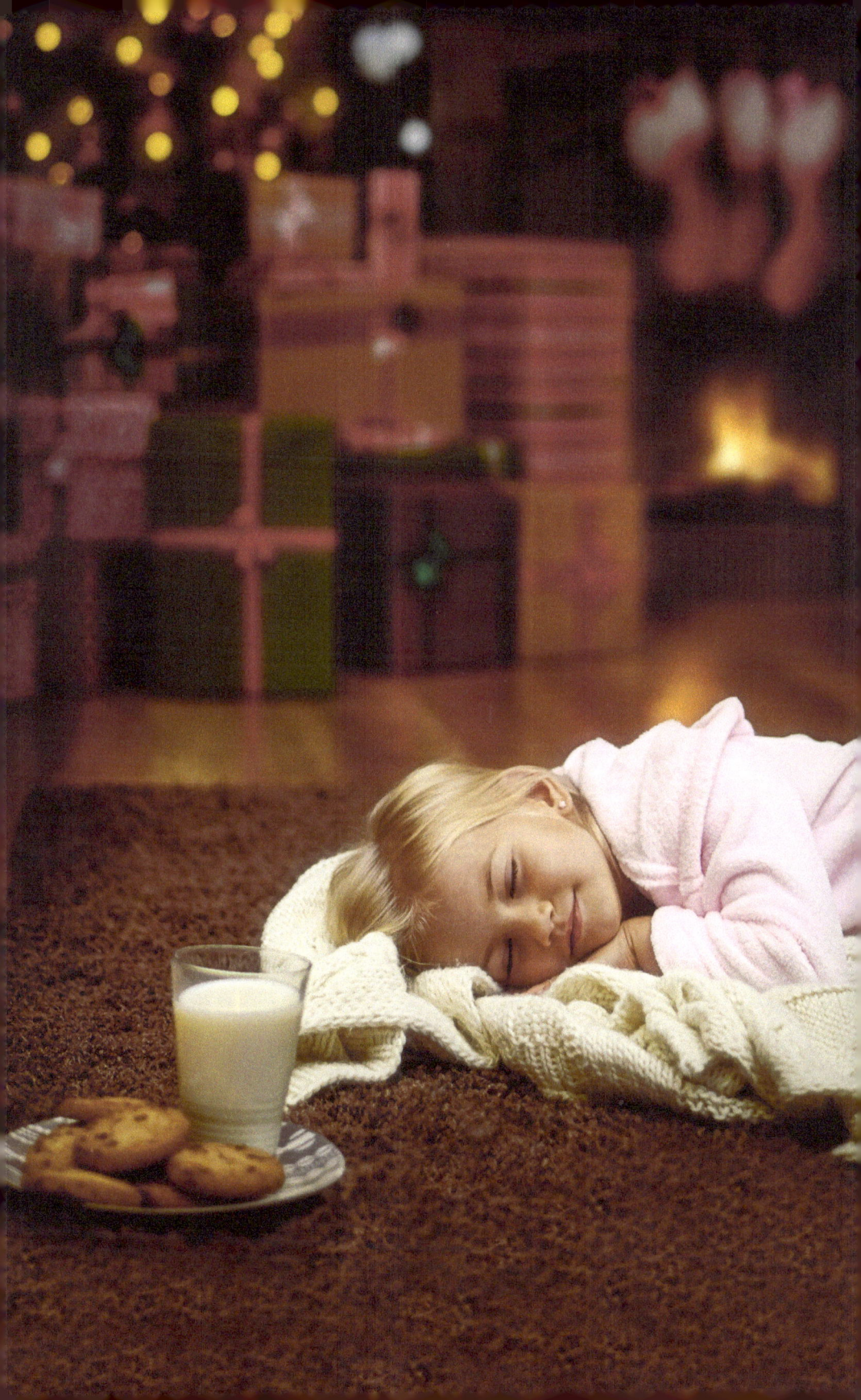

"One year my family spent Christmas at a cabin in Colorado. A heavy winter storm left us snowed in, but we didn't care. We had everything we needed for a perfect Christmas day, including the most delicious Christmas dinner ever."

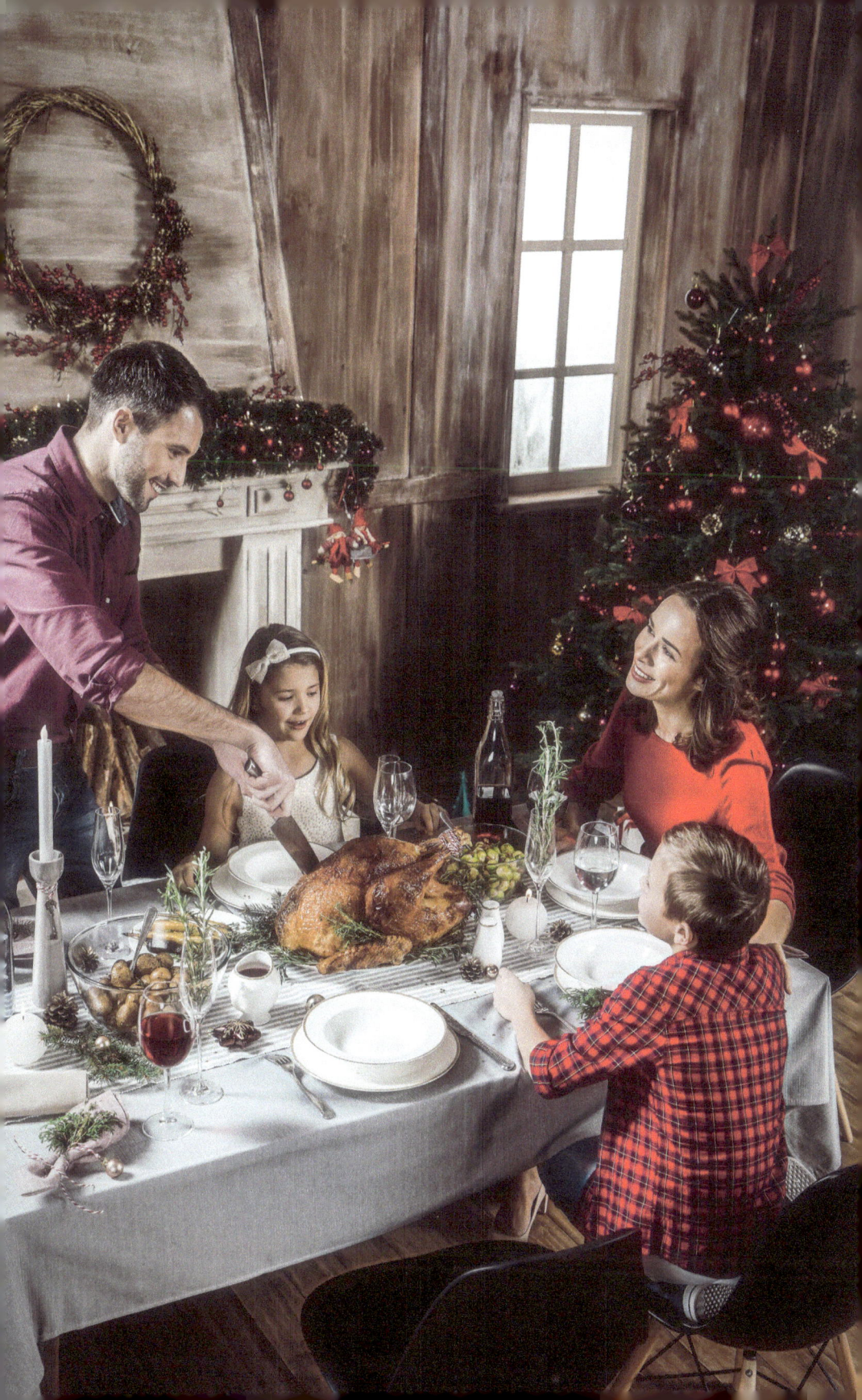

www.ingramcontent.com/pod-product-compliance
Lightning Source LLC
Chambersburg PA
CBHW040337220526
45473CB00009B/2714